W9-DGJ-361

PRAYERS FOR
HEALTH
AND
HEALING

—◦—

2000
The Continuum International Publishing Group Inc
370 Lexington Avenue
New York, NY 10017

Printed in the United Kingdom

Library of Congress Cataloguing-in-Publication Data

Prayers for health and healing
        p. cm.
ISBN 0-8264-1264-5
   1.   Sick—Prayer-books and devotions—English. I. Continuum (Firm)

 BV270 .P73 2000
   242'.861—dc21

                                                        00-024084

PRAYERS FOR
HEALTH
AND
HEALING

CONTINUUM • NEW YORK

PRAYERS FOR
HEALTH
AND
HEALING

PRAYERS FOR
HEALTH
AND
HEALING

CONTINUUM • NEW YORK

2000
The Continuum International Publishing Group Inc
370 Lexington Avenue
New York, NY 10017

Printed in the United Kingdom

Library of Congress Cataloguing-in-Publication Data

Prayers for health and healing
        p. cm.
    ISBN 0-8264-1264-5
    1. Sick—Prayer-books and devotions—English. I. Continuum (Firm)

    BV270 .P73 2000
    242'.861—dc21

                                        00-024084

CONTENTS

PREFACE

Many of us have had the experience of visiting someone ill, coming to the moment when we ought to go, and thinking, 'What should I do or say now?' Would it help to say a prayer? But we do not really know how to frame one, or fear embarrassment if we make that suggestion, so we mumble something useless and leave.

In truth we often can do nothing more helpful than pray with our friend or loved one. They are longing for us to do just that, and it is only fear of incompetence which stands in the way of a beautiful three-way encounter – between the person who is ill, God and you. Such an encounter can benefit the sick person at every level, and be a great encouragement.

This book is offered as a way to find the words that can elude us at such times. In the hands of a minister visiting in hospital or at a bedside, or in the pocket of a Christian friend wanting to pray with someone who is ill, *Prayers for Health and Healing* can give an appropriate, beautiful, healing expression to our longing for the deeper wellbeing of our loved ones in sickness.

Most sections are as their titles in the contents list suggest, but the first two sections may need a little explanation. In the first, we have tried to give voice in prayer to the nature of health. Health is more than merely a state of physical wholeness. It includes spiritual, emotional and mental health, and a capacity for living at a pace and in a style which expresses our personhood and God's unique *shalom*. Unless we build on a foundation of health properly understood, our prayers for healing will be defective.

In the second section, prayers for healing are drawn from several differing traditions of healing ministry. Some are in the form of brief liturgies; some involve anointing with oil; some come as close as written prayers can to the atmosphere of Spirit-directed prayer. Whatever your approach, it is intended that you find prayers you can use comfortably.

May this anthology of prayers strengthen your ministry and fellowship with the sick, and lead to some of those encounters with God and with others which can enrich everyone.

A Healthy Life

Psalm 23

The LORD is my shepherd, I shall
    not want.
  He makes me lie down in green
    pastures;
he leads me beside still waters;
  he restores my soul.
He leads me in right paths
  for his name's sake.

Even though I walk through the
    darkest valley,
  I fear no evil;
for you are with me;
  your rod and your staff—
  they comfort me.

You prepare a table before me
  in the presence of my enemies;
you anoint my head with oil;
  my cup overflows.
Surely goodness and mercy
  shall follow me
  all the days of my life,
and I shall dwell in the house of
    the LORD
  my whole life long.

2

Drop thy still dews of quietness,
   Till all our strivings cease;
Take from our souls the strain and stress,
   And let out ordered lives confess
     The beauty of thy peace.

Breathe through the heats of our desire
   Thy coolness and thy balm;
Let sense be dumb, let flesh retire;
Speak through the earthquake, wind, and fire,
     O still small voice of calm!

John Greenleaf Whittier

---

3   Slow me down, Lord! Ease the pounding of my heart by the quieting of my mind. Steady my hurried pace with a vision of the eternal reach of time. Give me amidst the confusion of my day the calmness of the everlasting hills. Allow me to know the magical restoring power of sleep. Teach me the art of taking one-minute vacations . . . of slowing down to look at a flower, to pat a dog, to read a few lines from a good book. Let me look up into the branches of the towering oak and know that it grew great and strong because it grew slowly and well.

   Slow me down Lord, and inspire me to send my roots deep into the soil of life's enduring values that I may grow toward the stars of my greater destiny.

Toc H

God, lovegiver,
    the love that dares to speak out,
    the love that listens,
    the love found most powerfully in weakness,
    the love that heals,
this is the love we need and long for,
not counterfeit pretty love, tied with bows,
but lasting love;
love that's there when the sweetness has gone;
love that endures beyond the barrier of pain.

Forgive us
    for worshipping the idols of perfection,
    for failing to see your glory in the vulnerable,
    for attaching more worth to the seen
    than the unseen,
    for being so full of our own importance
    that we cannot do the one thing needful.
        Lord, have mercy.
        Christ, have mercy.

Forgive us
    our lack of perseverance
    in face of failure, doubt, rejection;
    our failure to make connections
    between politics and health,
    economics and healing.
        Lord, have mercy.
        Christ, have mercy.

    Vulnerable lovegiver,
    Christ, wounded healer,
    Holy Spirit, compassionate friend,
    grant us love in all its fullness.

Kate McIlhagga

Psalm 103

Bless the LORD, O my soul,
  and all that is within me,
  bless his holy name.
Bless the LORD, O my soul,
  and do not forget all his
    benefits—
who forgives all your iniquity,
  who heals all your diseases,
who redeems your life from the
  Pit,
  who crowns you with steadfast
    love and mercy,
who satisfies you with good as
  long as you live
  so that your youth is renewed
    like the eagle's.

The LORD works vindication
  and justice for all who are
    oppressed.
He made known his ways to
    Moses,
  his acts to the people of Israel.
The LORD is merciful and
    gracious,
  slow to anger and abounding in
    steadfast love.
He will not always accuse,
  nor will he keep his anger
    forever.

He does not deal with us
according to our sins,
nor repay us according to our
iniquities.
For as the heavens are high above
the earth,
so great is his steadfast love
toward those who fear him;
as far as the east is from the west,
so far he removes our
transgressions from us.
As a father has compassion for his
children,
so the LORD has compassion for
those who fear him.
For he knows how we were made;
he remembers that we are dust.

As for mortals, their days are like
grass;
they flourish like a flower of the
field;
for the wind passes over it, and it
is gone,
and its place knows it no more.
But the steadfast love of the LORD
is from everlasting to
everlasting
on those who fear him,
and his righteousness to
children's children,
to those who keep his covenant
and remember to do his
commandments.

The LORD has established his
throne in the heavens,
and his kingdom rules over all.
Bless the LORD, O you his angels,
you mighty ones who do his
bidding,
obedient to his spoken word.
Bless the LORD, all his hosts,
his ministers that do his will.
Bless the LORD, all his works,
in all places of his dominion.
Bless the LORD, O my soul.

6

O Lord, give us yourself above all things.
It is in your coming alone that we are enriched.
It is in your coming that your true gifts come.
Come, Lord, that we may share the gifts of your presence.
Come, Lord, with healing of the past,
Come and calm our memories,
Come with joy for the present,
Come and give life to our existence,
Come with hope for the future,
Come and give a sense of eternity.
Come with strength for our wills,
Come with power for our thoughts,
Come with love for our heart,
Come and give affection to our being.
Come, Lord, give yourself above all things
And help us to give ourselves to you.

David Adam

I thank thee, God, that I have lived
In this great world and known its many joys:
The song of birds, the strong, sweet scent of hay
And cooling breezes in the secret dusk.
The flaming sunsets at the close of day,
Hills and the lonely, heather-covered moors,
Music at night and moonlight on the sea,
The beat of waves upon the rocky shore
And wild, white spray, flung high in ecstasy.
The faithful eyes of dogs and treasured books,
The love of kin and the fellowship of friends,
And all that makes life dear and beautiful.
I thank thee too, that there has come to me
A little sorrow and sometimes defeat,
A little heartache and the loneliness
That comes with parting, and the word 'Goodbye',
Dawn breaking after dreary hours of pain,
When I discovered that night's gloom must yield
And morning light break through to me again.
Because of these and other blessings poured
Unasked upon my wondering head,
Because I know that there is yet to come
An even richer and more glorious life,
And most of all, because thine only Son
Once sacrificed Life's loveliness for me –
I thank thee God that I have lived.

Elizabeth Craven

8 Dear God, it is so hard for us not to be anxious.
We worry about work and money,
about food and health,
about weather and crops,
about war and politics,
about loving and being loved.
Show us how perfect love casts out fear.

Monica Furlong

———⊃⊂———

9 I weave a silence to my lips,
my mind,
my heart.
Calm me, O Lord,
as you stilled the storm.
Still me, O Lord,
keep me from harm.
Let all the tumult
within me cease.
Enfold me, Lord,
in your peace.

Peter Millar, based on a Gaelic prayer

———⊃⊂———

10 Almighty God, who knowest our necessities before we ask, and our
ignorance in asking: set free thy servants from all anxious thought
for the morrow; give us contentment with thy good gifts; and con-
firm our faith that according as we seek thy kingdom, thou wilt not
suffer us to lack any good thing; through Jesus Christ our Lord.

Augustine of Hippo

———⊃⊂———

Arise, O sun of righteousness, upon us, with healing in thy wings; 11
make us children of the light and of the day. Show us the way in
which we should walk, for unto thee, O Lord, do we lift up our
souls. Dispel all mists of ignorance which cloud our understandings.
Let no false suggestion either withdraw our hearts from the love of
thy truth, or from the practice of it in all the actions of our lives; for
the sake of Jesus Christ our Lord.

Thomas Sherlock

Father, I give you thanks for all those times when you have been 12
with me in moments of weakness and suffering. More than ever
before, your love seemed all about me and beneath me. I remember
with gratitude the encouragement of friends and the care of those
who were closest to me. May the remembrance of your goodness
fill all the coming days with confidence and with hope.

More Everyday Prayers

O God, from whom to be turned is to fall, 13
to whom to be turned is to rise,
and in whom to stand is to abide for ever;
grant us in all our duties thy help,
in all our perplexities thy guidance,
in all our dangers thy protection,
and in all our sorrows thy peace;
through Jesus Christ our Lord.

Augustine of Hippo

Psalm 139

Where can I go from your spirit?
    Or where can I flee from your
        presence?
If I ascend to heaven, you are
        there;
    if I make my bed in Sheol, you
        are there.
If I take the wings of the morning
    and settle at the farthest limits
        of the sea,
even there your hand shall lead
        me,
    and your right hand shall hold
        me fast.
If I say, 'Surely the darkness shall
        cover me,
    and the light around me become
        night,'
even the darkness is not dark to
        you;
    the night is as bright as the day,
    for darkness is as light to you.

For it was you who formed my
        inward parts;
    you knit me together in my
        mother's womb.
I praise you, for I am fearfully and
        wonderfully made.
    Wonderful are your works;
that I know very well.
    My frame was not hidden from
        you,
when I was being made in secret,

> intricately woven in the depths
>   of the earth.
> Your eyes beheld my unformed
>   substance.
> In your book were written
>   all the days that were formed
>   for me,
>   when none of them as yet
>   existed.
> How weighty to me are your
>   thoughts, O God!
>   How vast is the sum of them!
> I try to count them—they are
>   more than the sand;
>   I come to the end—I am still
>   with you.

———◦———

Give me a candle of the Spirit, O God, as I go down into the deeps   15
of my being. Show me the hidden things, the creatures of my
dreams, the storehouse of forgotten memories and hurts. Take me
down to the spring of my life, and tell me my nature and my name.
Give me freedom to grow, so that I may become that self, the seed
of which you planted in me at my making. Out of the deeps I cry
to you, O God.

George Appleton

———◦———

16   Almighty and merciful God, who art the strength of the weak, the refreshment of the weary, the comfort of the sad, the help of the tempted, the life of the dying, the God of patience and of all consolation; thou knowest full well the inner weakness of our nature, how we tremble and quiver before pain, and cannot bear the cross without thy divine help and support. Help me, then, O eternal and pitying God, help me to possess my soul in patience, to maintain unshaken hope in thee, to keep that childlike trust which feels a Father's heart hidden beneath the cross; so shall I be strengthened with power according to thy glorious might, in all patience and long-suffering; I shall be enabled to endure pain and temptation, and, in the very depth of my suffering, to praise thee with a joyful heart.

Johann Habermann

17   O Great Caregiver,
bring good health to the growing,
good sense to the striving,
good soul to the searching.
O Great Caregiver,
bring clarity to the mind,
charity to the heart,
strength to the body,
so we may serve you well.

Lisa Withrow

Eternal God and Father, help us to entrust the past to your mercy,   18
the present to your love, and the future to your wisdom, in the
name of Jesus Christ our Lord, who is the same yesterday, and today,
and for ever.

Source unknown

⸺⸺

Creator and Ruler of heaven and earth,   19
    the universe is in the palm of your hand.

You sent your Son to give us life,
    life in all its fullness
    living water
    bread eternal.

Enable us to live as you willed in the beginning,
    washed in him,
    fed by him,
that we may enter into that wholeness and salvation
    which comes from you.

In your goodness, Lord, hear us.

John Gunstone

⸺⸺

Psalm 91

You who live in the shelter of the
    Most High,
  who abide in the shadow of the
    Almighty,
will say to the LORD, 'My refuge
    and my fortress;
  my God, in whom I trust.'
For he will deliver you from the
    snare of the fowler
  and from the deadly pestilence;
he will cover you with his
    pinions,
  and under his wings you will
    find refuge;
  his faithfulness is a shield and
    buckler.
You will not fear the terror of the
    night,
  or the arrow that flies by day,
or the pestilence that stalks in
    darkness,
  or the destruction that wastes at
    noonday.

A thousand may fall at your side,
    ten thousand at your right hand,
  but it will not come near you.
You will only look with your eyes
  and see the punishment of the
    wicked.

Because you have made the LORD
  your refuge,

the Most High your dwelling
      place,
no evil shall befall you,
      no scourge come near your tent.

For he will command his angels
      concerning you
      to guard you in all your ways.
On their hands they will bear you
      up,
      so that you will not dash your
      foot against a stone.
You will tread on the lion and the
      adder,
      the young lion and the serpent
      you will trample under
      foot.

Those who love me, I will deliver;
      I will protect those who know
      my name.
When they call to me, I will
      answer them;
      I will be with them in trouble,
      I will rescue them and honour
      them.
With long life I will satisfy
      them,
      and show them my salvation.

21
Once life has almost been
taken from you,
When for some strange reason
you emerge from death
and blink
with new eyes upon the old
almost forgotten universe,
then you can understand
once more
the value of sea and stars,
of happiness uncontainable,
the sheer relief and delight of being alive
that turns your eyes repeatedly
upwards
with thanksgiving
then straight outward
declaring peace over and over again
to those who with heads bent low
see mud not stars.

Kathy Keay

22
We thank you, gracious God,
that we are the guests at your table.
As we have been fed by your gifts of life,
so we will share with the world
all that you give to us in love.

Dorothy McRae-McMahon

Most heavenly Father of the human race, behold me, unworthy   23
though I am; see that I am about to have a baby. I pray that you assist
me to bear the pain of childbirth courageously, and give me physical and moral strength. Avert from me any unseen or unnatural
circumstance and grant me the privilege of bearing a normal,
healthy baby. Hear my humble prayer, dear Lord, offered to you
with confidence and love in this hour of my expectation. Help me
to be a good mother in word and example. Grant that after my
delivery my little baby may learn at an early age of your greatness.
May the joy and peace of a safe delivery fill my heart, and may your
blessed name be praised now and for evermore.

Sister E. Gbonda

⸺◁▷⸺

O God, thank you for the joy of a new baby in our family, for a new   24
life which is part of us and yet a separate being. As we love and care
for our child help us to teach him/her to know and love you as
his/her friend.

Chelmsford diocese, England

⸺◁▷⸺

Prayers for Healing

THE WITNESS

Leader   In Jesus Christ, we hear the Good News
that God is like a mother hen
who shelters her chickens
under her warm wings.

People   **We believe that God is love.**

Leader   In Jesus, we see a God
who wept for the people of the world,

People   **and weeps for our wounding.**

Leader   In Jesus, we see a God
who reaches out with healing hands,

People   **who sees our pain and makes us whole.**

CONFESSION

Leader   Let us join in our prayers of confession:
O God, you die for us and conquer death for us,

People   **but we find it hard to believe in your love.**

Leader   We see your creativity in all the earth,

People   **but fear to ask for our own healing.**

All   **Forgive us and bring us to faith.**

ASSURANCE OF PARDON

Leader   Hear the word to us in Christ:
If we have faith as small as a mustard seed,
God's power is released in us.
Our healing is a gracious gift.
Rise, take up your bed and walk.
Amen.

People   **Amen.**

PRAYERS OF INTERCESSION

Leader   O God, we cry to you in our anger
            that people hurt each other.

People   **Be with us and heal us, O God.**

Leader   We feel the fear and pain
            of an innocent and trusting child.

People   **Be with us and heal us, O God.**

Leader   We carry with us the things
            that have been done to us
            which hurt and destroy.

People   **Be with us and heal us, O God.**

Leader   They stand before us
            and weigh us down.
            They stop us living with joy and hope.

People   **Be with us and heal us, O God.**

Leader   Lift us up
            on the wings of your Spirit.

People   **Set us free with your peace
            and your power.**

Leader   For you are stronger
            than all the forces that stand against us.

People   **Set us free,
            heal our wounds,
            O God who never leaves us
            nor forsakes us.
            Amen.**

THE LAYING OF HANDS

(The person seeking healing kneels.)

Minister   We lay our hands upon you
              in the name of Jesus Christ,

24

healer and lover of the world.

(Silent prayer)

May the Lord of love,
who is more powerful
than all those who would harm us,
give you healing for all that is past
and peace for all that is to come.
May she surround you
with comfort and warmth
and fill you with life
that is stronger than death.

People   **Amen.**

THE ANOINTING

Minister   Lift your face to the light.
You are beautiful in the sight of God.
The mark of Christ is upon you;
walk free and open your heart to life,
for Christ walks with you
into a new day.

People   **Amen.**

Dorothy McRae-McMahon

26   Healer of the ages,
       we lift our loved one to you
       for healing – in body, mind and spirit.
       May we open our hearts to possibility
       may we know your presence in this place
       may we find courage and strength to trust
       in your name.

       Prayer for Cleansing
       Almighty One,
           we approach you in quiet awe
           we approach you seeking health
           we pray for faith to trust
           we pray for forgiveness
           we pray for cleansing of thought, word and deed.
       Make us ready to receive you
       in this holy place.

       We give thanks for your anointing
       of the ill and the troubled.
       Purify us so that we may receive
       this oil of healing.
       Pour out your Holy Spirit upon us
       and upon this gift
       so that we may be made whole in your name.

Anointing with oil (participants may want to touch one hoping for healing, if appropriate)

       Leader (making sign of the cross on forehead or hands or both)
               Child of God, I anoint you with oil, in the name of
               the holy and triune God, Creator and Healer of
               all things.

Those laying hands on person's head or hand
> These hands are laid on you, in the name of the
> holy and triune God, Creator and Healer of all
> things.

Leader May the power of God heal you
> in body
> in mind
> in spirit
> in relationship.
> So be it.

Prayer of Thanksgiving
> We are grateful, all-knowing One
> for your gifts here today.
> Let us know your peace now
> and live in gratitude
> for the promise of your presence.

Blessing
> The God who heals you
> bless and keep you.
> The God who knows you
> grant you deep peace.

Lisa Withrow

27

27 OPENING SENTENCES

Leader   Our God is a God who longs to be with us

People   **Who reaches into our deepest places**
who weeps within our tears.

Leader   Our God is a God who holds us
in the womb-space of compassion

People   **Labouring to bring us to birth**
in the new life of freedom,
tasting the blood of our pain.

Leader   Our God is like a rock

People   **Unmoved from love,**
unshaken by the anger in our righteous protest
firm beneath our feet
in the eternal creating of our holy ground.

THE GRIEVING JOURNEY

Leader   Let us recall the journey of grieving,
the place of safety and joy which has been left
and the loss along the way.

(The grievings, losses and disappointments are named.)

THE AFFIRMATION

All   **There is no death**
from which you cannot rise in us,
O God.
The power to fail
can never kill the gift of life,
unless we choose
not to receive it from you.
Your Spirit is never defeated
by the woundings of life

however unjust,
however painful.
Your grace in Christ
goes well beyond our understanding
and your love for us
is never measured
by our love for ourselves.
Even as we walk a hard journey
we will claim together
this great hope.
Amen.

PRAYERS OF INTERCESSION

Leader   Let us place in the hands of God,
          all that disturbs us,
          all our longings for those whom we hold
          in loving concern:

          (The people share their prayers.)

Leader   O Lord, hear our prayer.

THE ANOINTING

Leader   In the name of the Christ,
          who has walked every journey before you
          and sees deeply into your heart in understanding,
          we announce a new day.
          Receive the grace of God
          and the healing of the Holy Spirit,
          in the name of Christ,

All   **Amen.**

          (The people pass to each other a pot of fragrant oil and anoint
          each other on the hand or forehead with the words 'Receive the
          grace of God.')

29

BLESSING

Leader   Go in peace.
And may the God of grace encircle your soul
the God in Christ reach out to touch you
and the Spirit shine light on your path.

All   **Amen.**

Dorothy McRae-McMahon

———⊃⊂———

28   *At an anointing*

As outwardly and with sacramental oil
your body is anointed
so may Almighty God, our Father,
inwardly anoint your soul, to strengthen you
with all the comfort and the joy
of his most Holy Spirit,
and to loose you from all that troubles you
in body, mind, or spirit.
May he send you forth,
renewed and restored to do his will,
to your benefit, in the service of others.
but above all to the glory of his Holy Name.

*Prayer used at the
church of St Marylebone*

———⊃⊂———

Jesus, our Lord and Shepherd,
  you had compassion on the weak and disabled
    the two blind beggars
    the crippled at Bethesda,
    the deaf, the dumb,
    the mentally ill,
    and those troubled by evil spirits.

By the anointing of your Spirit
  bring comfort, peace and healing
    to . . . in his distress.
May he have patience to accept what cannot be changed
  and faith to receive the healing which you offer him
    in body, mind and spirit.

Equip us with discernment and love
  to encourage him to respond to you,
    to the honour and glory of the heavenly Father.

John Gunstone

———⊃⊂———

    At even ere the sun was set,
    The sick, O Lord, around thee lay;
    Oh, in what divers pains they met!
    Oh, with what joy they went away!

    Thy touch has still its ancient power;
    No word from thee can fruitless fall;
    Hear, in this solemn evening hour,
    And in thy mercy heal us all.

    H. Twells

———⊃⊂———

31 Lord, at this moment . . . is desperately ill. May they be calmed and comforted by the knowledge that your merciful eyes are watching them. May they get relief during the long, sleepless hours of night and relief from their pain. If it be your will, restore them to health and strength, and comfort all those who watch and wait.

Brenda Thorpe

32   I am praying for my friend who is so very ill.
O my Lord, you brought the touch of healing
to those who crossed your path
in your earthly life.
You promised to respond to the prayers
of your children that struggle to follow
and reflect you on this earth.
Reach out now to this one with your healing touch.
She belongs to you, O God.
She yearns so deeply to serve you.
Restore her to life and wholeness once more.
And even while she suffers,
may she sense your nearness
and be embraced by your peace.
Grant that she may have joy
even in the midst of her sufferings.
And grant, blessed Lord,
that she might get well again.

Leslie F. Brandt

You, who said, 'Come unto me all ye who are weary and heavy-laden and I will give you rest,' I come to you now. 33

For I am weary indeed. Mentally and physically I am bone-tired. I am all wound up, locked up tight with tension. I am too tired to eat. Too tired to think. Too tired even to sleep. I feel close to the point of exhaustion.

Lord, let your healing love flow through me.

I can feel it easing my tensions. Thank you. I can feel my body relaxing. Thank you. I can feel my mind begin to go calm and quiet and composed.

Thank you for unwinding me, Lord, for unlocking me. I am no longer tight and frozen with tiredness, but flowing freely, softly, gently into your healing rest.

Marjorie Holmes

—◦◦—

Jesus our Saviour, 34
    make yourself known to me
        as I enter the hospital.
Help me to adjust to this new manner of life.
Give me gratitude for those who care for me,
        compassion for those in the ward with me,
            and love for them all.

John Gunstone

—◦◦—

35   O Christ our Lord,
As in times past,
Not all the sick and suffering
Found their own way to your side,
But had to have their hands taken,
   or their bodies carried,
   or their names mentioned;
So we, confident of your goodness,
Bring others to you.

As in times past,
You looked at the faith of friends
and let peace and healing be known,
Look on our faith,
Even our little faith,
And let your kingdom come.

We name before you
Those for whom pain is the greatest problem;
Who are remembered more for their distress
   than for their potential;
Who at night cry, 'I wish to God it were morning.'
And in the morning cry, 'I wish to God it were night' . . .
Bring healing, bring peace.

We name before you
Those whose problem is not physical;
Those who are haunted by the nightmares of their past
   or the spectres of their future,
Those whose minds are shackled to neuroses,
   depression and fears,
Who do not know what is wrong
And do not know what to pray . . .

Lord Jesus Christ, Lover of all,
Bring healing, bring peace.

We name before you
Those in whose experience light has turned to darkness,
As the end of a life
Or the breaking of a relationship
Leaves them stunned in their souls
    and silent in their conversation,
Not knowing where to turn or who to turn to
or whether life has a purpose any more . . .

Lord Jesus Christ, Lover of all
Bring healing, bring peace.

And others whose troubles we do not know
Or whose names we would not say aloud,
We mention now in the silence which you understand . . .

Lord Jesus Christ, Lover of all
Bring healing, bring peace.

Lord God,
You alone are skilled to know the cure
For every sickness and every soul.
If by our lives your grace may be known
Then in us, through us,
And, if need be, despite us,
Let your kingdom come.

On all who tend the sick,
    counsel the distressed,
    sit with the dying,
    or develop medical research
We ask your blessing,
That in caring for your people
They may meet and serve their Lord.

And for those who, in this land,
Administer the agencies of health and welfare,
We ask your guidance that in all they do
Human worth may be valued,
And the service of human need fully resourced.
This we ask in the name of him
Whose flesh and blood have made all God's children special.

John Bell (Iona Community)

36

May your healing touch be with one
    who suffered.
May your new life be with one
    who died.
For Christ knew the meaning of suffering,
and Christ died, and came to live again.

May your healing touch be with us
    who suffer.
May your new life be with us
    who grieve.
For Christ knew the meaning of suffering,
and Christ can bring us hope again.

Lisa Withrow

May God who made you make you whole
as he would have you be,
in the name and through the power
of the Risen and Ascended Christ,
present with us now in his Holy Spirit.
May he send you forth,
renewed and restored to do his will,
to your benefit, in the service of others,
but above all to the glory of his Holy Name.

37

*Prayer used at the
church of St Marylebone*

Lord,
    I come to you in penitence,
        in trust, in hope:
I come praising your glorious name.

Heal every part of me, in body,
    in mind, in spirit.
Save me from all evil.

For I long to serve you, in joy,
    in peace and in power,
and to praise you all my days.

38

John Gunstone

39   Helper of all who are helpless,
we call on you in times of stress
and in times of devastation.
Pick up the broken pieces
of our hearts, our homes, our history
and restore them to the way they were,
or give us the means of starting over
when everything seems lost.
O God, our help in ages past,
we place all our hope in you.

Miriam Therese Winter

40   Father, give to us, and to all your people, in times of anxiety, serenity; in times of hardship, courage; in times of uncertainty, patience; and, at all times, a quiet trust in your wisdom and love; through Jesus Christ our Lord.

New Every Morning

41   We humbly beseech thee, of thy goodness, O Lord, to comfort and succour all them who in this transitory life are in trouble, sorrow, need, sickness, or any other adversity: help us to minister to them thy strength and consolation, and so endow us with the grace of sympathy and compassion that we may bring to them both help and healing; through Jesus Christ our Lord.

Church of England. Book of Common Prayer

Lord of the Universe   42
look in love upon your people.
Pour the healing oil of your compassion
on a world that is wounded and dying.
Send us out in search of the lost,
to comfort the afflicted,
to bind up the broken,
and to free those trapped
under the rubble of their fallen dreams.

Sheila Cassidy

＜○＞

As the body fights for life   43
as the mind fights for life
as the soul fights for life
may your healing touch be here.

As the days remain uncertain
as the nights lie dark and long
as dear ones become more precious
may your healing touch be here.

In the days of shadows
in the nights
in all time
may your healing touch bless this one,
may your boundless love know this one,
may your steadfast peace grace this one,
in all ways, in all ways.

Lisa Withrow

＜○＞

44   God of all consolation,
you chose and sent your Son to heal the world.
Graciously listen to our prayer of faith:
send the power of your Holy Spirit, the Consoler,
into this precious oil, this soothing ointment,
this rich gift, the fruit of the earth.

Bless this oil (+) and sanctify it for our use.

Make this oil a remedy for all who are anointed
    with it;
heal them in body, in soul, and in spirit,
and deliver them from every affliction.
We ask this through our Lord Jesus Christ, your
    Son, who lives
and reigns with you and the Holy Spirit, one God,
    for ever and ever.

John Gunstone

45   God, with your healing, anoint this one who suffers
God, with your ease, bless this one who feels pain
God, with your promise, come upon this one who searches
God, with your strength, breathe upon this one who labours.

A healing touch
a word of ease
a breath of promise
a gift of strength.
These things we ask of you, long-suffering one, this day.

Lisa Withrow

Prayers for
Doctors, Nurses, Carers

Dearest Lord, may I see you today and every day in the person of   46
your sick, and whilst nursing minister to you.

Though you hide yourself behind the unattractive disguise of the irritable, the exacting, the unreasonable, may I still recognize you and say: 'Jesus, my patient, how sweet it is to serve you.'

Lord, give me this seeing faith, then my work will never be monotonous. I will ever find joy in humouring the fancies and gratifying the wishes of all poor sufferers.

O beloved sick, how doubly dear you are to me, when you personify Christ; and what a privilege is mine to be allowed to tend you.

Sweetest Lord, make me appreciative of the dignity of my high vocation, and its many responsibilities. Never permit me to disgrace it by giving way to coldness, unkindness, or impatience.

And, O God, while you are Jesus, my patient, deign also to be to me a patient Jesus, bearing with my faults, looking only to my intention, which is to love and serve you in the person of each of your sick.

Lord, increase my faith, bless my efforts and work, now and for evermore.

Prayer offered daily by Mother Teresa's helpers in Shishu Bhavan, Calcutta

———✠———

God our Father, whose son, Jesus Christ, loved to bring health and   47
healing to those who were ill, may the Holy Spirit help and teach all doctors so that they try to find out more and more about curing and preventing illness. And help them too always to do their work lovingly and patiently even when they are very tired, just as Jesus did. Father, hear our prayer, for his sake.

Hope Freeman

———✠———

48   Almighty God, who calledst Luke the Physician, whose praise is in the Gospel, to be an Evangelist, and Physician of the soul: May it please thee that, by the wholesome medicines of the doctrine delivered by him, all the diseases of our souls may be healed; through the merits of thy Son Jesus Christ our Lord. Amen.

Collect for the feast of St Luke, Book of Common Prayer

49   Loving Father,
      I put myself into your hands.
  Deliver me from fear of pain and of the unknown.
  Set the cross of your dear Son over me,
     and guide with your wise Spirit
       the surgeon, the anaesthetist,
  and the theatre staff.
  Anoint them as servants of your healing power,
     and while I am unconscious
       may my deepest thoughts and feelings rest
        in you.
  May I sleep in your peace
     and awake to praise your mercy and your glory.

John Gunstone

Lord, we thank you for the great resources of healing that are available to those who are sick. 50

For the skill of surgeons and the technical abilities of support staff in operating theatres,
thank you.

For medical knowledge and the healing power of drugs and medicines,
for chemists and pharmacists,
thank you.

For nursing staff, for their professional skill and their capacity for caring and encouraging,
thank you.

For support teams of physiotherapists, occupational therapists, radiologists, hospital social workers and hospital chaplains,
thank you.

For administrative staff, ward orderlies, hospital porters and ambulance drivers,
thank you.

Further Everyday Prayers

47

51   Bless, O Lord Christ, all whom you have called to share in your
own ministry of healing as doctors and nurses. Give them skill,
understanding and compassion; and enable them to do their work
in dependence on your grace and for the promotion of your glory.

Mothers Union, United Kingdom

52   Lord Jesus, who healed the sick and gave them new life, be with
doctors and nurses as they act as agents of your healing touch. In
desperate times keep them strong yet loving and, when their work
is done, be with them in their tears as they share with parents the
sorrow of losing a child.

Althea Hayton

53   Loving Lord Jesus, you spent much of your time on earth healing
sick bodies and bringing health to troubled minds. Bless, we pray
you, all those who are continuing your work in clinics and hospitals throughout the world. In your name we ask it.

Joyce Care

Thank you, O God, for all the people who have looked after me 54
today; for all those who visited today; for all the letters and the get-
well cards; for the flowers and gifts friends have sent.

I know that sleep is one of the best medicines for both the body
and the mind. Help me to sleep tonight.

Into your strong hands I place all the patients in this ward; the
night staff on duty tonight; my loved ones, whose names I now
mention; myself, with my fears, my worries and my hopes.

Help me to sleep, thinking of you and your promises.

Source unknown

Lord Jesus Christ, we ask you to be with all those who need your 55
healing touch today. Come in all your power and surround them
with your love. Bless the work of our hospitals, health centres, day
centres, the hospice movement, the Samaritans and all those who
seek to ease the pain and anxieties of the sick.

Julie Densham

Lord, we thank you for the hospice movement. We pray for your 56
blessing on the hospices in the cities and towns of our land. Guide
all who administer them; give wisdom to those who counsel
patients and their families, and gentleness and patience to those
who nurse the sick and dying.

May all be ready to bring quietness, peace and preparation for the
life to come to those in their care. Through Jesus Christ our Lord.

Mary Batchelor

57   Jesus, you cared for all the sick
      who came to you.
   I want to care with loving compassion,
      to attend to details with gentleness.
   But I become weary and impatient,
      angry and abrupt.
   It is hard to watch the suffering of someone I love,
      hard to find energy for all I must do.
   I grow discouraged and resentful.
   Let me learn from your life of compassion.
Spirit of healing and comfort,
   Be with me in these difficult times.
   Teach me to take time for myself,
      to be gentle with my own limits,
      to ask for help from others.
   May your grace allow me
      to forgive myself when I fail,
      to let go of my expectations,
      to grieve all my losses.
   Send your healing power to me and the one for
      whom I care. We trust in your love.

Kathleen Fischer

————⋯————

Lord, your touch has still its healing power. Here are my hands: take 58
them and use them this day in humble service so that your love may
flow through them to someone who needs a human touch.

Sheila King

Loving Lord, 59
time can only heal
provided I'm willing to take time
to realise that I have within my human mystery
the seeds of becoming a wounded healer.
By taking my own brokenness on board
and living with, in and through it
I gradually notice new strengths developing.
By giving my own wounds an airing
And letting them have breathing space,
I'm slowly but surely making more room for others
in their woundedness.
By feeling my own powerlessness
I begin to let a power greater than myself
have room and scope to work in me.

Lord of my memory and my memories,
let me let you heal me.

Althea Hayton

60 Grant us grace, O Father, not to pass by suffering or joy without eyes to see. Give us understanding and sympathy, and guard us from selfishness, that we may enter into the joys and sufferings of others. Use us to gladden and strengthen those who are weak and suffering; that by our lives we may help others to believe and serve thee, and shed forth thy light which is the light of life.

H. R. L. (Dick) Sheppard

61
In the name of the Healer,
bring strength to the carer,
in the name of the Healer
bring relief to the giver,
in the name of the Healer
bring courage to the carer,
in the name of the Healer
bring rest to the giver,
for you are the Giver of Care –
and in adversity, you are with us.

Lisa Withrow

62
You were despised and rejected of men, O Lord;
a man of sorrows and acquainted with grief,
so you can understand when I feel rejected;
you can feel my sorrow and my sadness.
I thank you for your presence
in all my times of darkness,
and for giving me light along my way.

Denis Duncan

Father, to you I raise my whole being,   63
A vessel emptied of self. Accept, Lord,
this my emptiness, and so fill me with
yourself – your light, love, and life –
that these your precious gifts may
radiate through me, and overflow
the chalice of my heart into
the hearts of all with
whom I come into
contact this day,
revealing to
them the beauty
of your joy and
wholeness,
and
the
serenity
of your peace,
which nothing can destroy.

Frances Nuttal

Enduring Pain and Suffering

Lord, look down on me in my infirmities   64
and help me to bear them patiently.

St Francis of Assisi

———⊃⊂———

Dear Jesus, when I woke up this morning my body ached all over.   65
I felt miserable and low in spirit, trying to cope with the pain and
sleeplessness of the night. I asked you, Jesus, to help me through
another day. Thank you that once more, Jesus, you heard and
answered my prayer.

Monmouth diocese, Wales

———⊃⊂———

Jesus, you know how tired I feel. Give me strength in my body. Let   66
your love and patience be with me, so that I will not speak in a cross
voice any words that may hurt. Help us both to love each other as
you love us.

Thank you, Jesus, for understanding the needs of us all. Thank
you for this day.

June Waters

———⊃⊂———

67
We call on strength
for one who lives day to day,
we call on strength
for one who suffers day to day,
we call on comfort
for one who fights illness,
we call on comfort
for one who fights despair,
we call on courage
for the future,
we call on courage
for the loved ones,
we call on love
for one who learns
to hope beyond all hope
for wholeness.

Lisa Withrow

68 Lord, we bring before you all who suffer, especially those whose ailments are concealed. Pour out upon them your healing love, we pray, and so strengthen their faith that they may be made whole. Grant to us the grace of consideration, that we be not impatient with uncomprehended handicaps.

Rochester diocese, England

Lord God, whose Son, Jesus Christ, understood people's fear and   69
pain before they spoke of them, we pray for those in hospital.
Surround the frightened with your tenderness; give strength to
those in pain; hold the weak in your arms of love; and give hope
and patience to those who are recovering. We ask this through the
same Jesus Christ, our Lord.

Christine McMullen

Depression and Sorrow

Psalm 22

My God, my God, why have you
    forsaken me?
  Why are you so far from
    helping me, from the
    words of my groaning?
O my God, I cry by day, but you
    do not answer;
  and by night, but find no rest.

Yet you are holy,
    enthroned on the praises of
    Israel.
In you our ancestors trusted;
    they trusted, and you delivered
    them.
To you they cried, and were
    saved;
    in you they trusted, and were
    not put to shame.

But I am a worm, and not human;
    scorned by others, and despised
    by the people.
All who see me mock at me;
    they make mouths at me, they
    shake their heads;
'Commit your cause to the LORD;
    let him deliver—
    let him rescue the one in whom
    he delights!'

Yet it was you who took me from
    the womb;
     you kept me safe on my
      mother's breast.
On you I was cast from my birth,
    and since my mother bore me
     you have been my God.
Do not be far from me,
    for trouble is near
    and there is no one to help.

Many bulls encircle me,
    strong bulls of Bashan surround
     me;
they open wide their mouths at
    me,
     like a ravening and roaring lion.

I am poured out like water,
    and all my bones are out of
     joint;
my heart is like wax;
    it is melted within my breast;
my mouth is dried up like a
    potsherd,
     and my tongue sticks to my
     jaws;
     you lay me in the dust of death.

For dogs are all around me;
    a company of evildoers encircles
     me.
My hands and feet have
    shrivelled;
I can count all my bones.
They stare and gloat over me;

64

they divide my clothes among
      themselves,
   and for my clothing they cast
      lots.

But you, O LORD, do not be far
      away!
   O my help, come quickly to my
      aid!
Deliver my soul from the sword,
   my life from the power of the
      dog!
   Save me from the mouth of the
      lion!

From the horns of the wild oxen
      you have rescued me.
I will tell of your name to my
      brothers and sisters;
   in the midst of the congregation
      I will praise you:
You who fear the LORD, praise
      him!
   All you offspring of Jacob,
      glorify him;
   stand in awe of him, all you
      offspring of Israel!
For he did not despise or abhor
   the affliction of the afflicted;
he did not hide his face from me,
   but heard when I cried to him.

71 Grant, O God, that amidst all the discouragements, difficulties and dangers, distress and darkness of this mortal life, I may depend upon thy mercy, and on this build my hopes, as on a sure foundation. Let thine infinite mercy in Christ Jesus deliver me from despair, both now and at the hour of death.

Thomas Wilson

72 God of love, you watch with all who weep or worry.
You offer hope to those in despair
and your calming presence to the troubled.
Give us peace.

Leta Hawe

73 As the rain hides the stars,
as the autumn mist hides the hills,
as the clouds veil the blue of the sky so the dark
happenings of my lot hide the shining of your face from me.

Yet if I may hold your hand in the darkness it is enough.
Since I know that though I may stumble in my going, you
do not fall.

Translated by Alistair Maclean

74

Lord, I am crushed by this sense of my
    unworthiness.
There is nothing in my life that I can call good.
  I despise myself.
  I loathe my thoughts and desires;
    they poison and corrupt me.
If others could look into my heart
    they would never want to know me again.

But you know me, Lord, intimately.
  In your incarnate life
you saw into the hearts of women and men;
    you discerned their secret faults.
There is nothing in me that is hidden from you.
    Yet you still love me,
      for you came to call sinners like me.
You are my Redeemer.

Lord, in your love, send cleansing fire into my
    innermost being.
Drive from me the spirits of self-hatred and
    depression,
    banish them so that they never trouble me again.
And fill me with your Spirit
    that I may grow in love for you and for others.

John Gunstone

75   Light of the world, it is hard to connect with you
when little has meaning for this one.
Send your light through the darkness
send your light to shine in despair
give energy to clear the inner angers.

Light of the world, help us connect with you
to find meaning for this one.
Send your light to bring meaning
send your light to bring focus
outside the walls of depression.

Stir life in your loved one,
stir inner purpose too.
Stir humour and lightness,
break through the walls of depression,
break through the walls.

Lisa Withrow

---

76   I have no other helper than you, no other father, I pray
      to you.
Only you can help me. My present misery is too great.
Despair grips me, and I am at my wit's end.
O Lord, Creator, Ruler of the World, Father,
I thank you that you have brought me through.
How strong the pain was – but you were stronger.
How deep the fall was – but you were even deeper.
How dark the night was – but you were the noonday
    sun in it.
You are our father, our mother, our brother, and our friend.

An African prayer

O Lord, Jesus Christ, Who art as the Shadow of a Great Rock in a 77
weary land, Who beholdest Thy weak creatures weary of labour,
weary of pleasure, weary of hope deferred, weary of self; in Thine
abundant compassion, and fellow-feeling with us, and unutterable
tenderness, bring us, we pray Thee, unto Thy rest.

Christina Rossetti

Father,   78
we pray for those
who know the suffering
of total despair:
for the terminally ill
and the grief-stricken;
for the depressed
and for those consumed by guilt;
for those who have lost their faith
in life, in others, in you.
We bring before you
those who feel totally alone
when faced with fears and pain
that threaten to overwhelm them.

Christine Odell

79

Lord, hear my prayer when trouble glooms,
Let sorrow find a way,
and when the day of trouble comes,
Turn not thy face away:
My bones like hearthstones burn away,
My life like vapoury smoke decays.

My heart is smitten like the grass,
That withered lies and dead,
And I, so lost to what I was,
Forget to eat my bread.
My voice is groaning all the day,
My bones prick through this skin of clay.

The wilderness' pelican,
The desert's lonely owl –
I am their like, a desert man
In ways as lone and foul.
As sparrows on the cottagetop
I wait till I with fainting drop.

I hear my enemies reproach,
All silently I mourn;
They on my private peace encroach,
Against me they are sworn.
Ashes as bread my trouble shares,
And mix my food with weeping cares.

Yet not for them is sorrow's toil,
I fear no mortal's frowns –
But thou hast held me up awhile
And thou has cast me down.
My days like shadows waste from view,
I mourn like withered grass in dew.

But thou, Lord, shalt endure for ever,
All generations through;
Thou shalt to Zion be the giver
Of joy and mercy too.
Her very stones are in thy trust,
·Thy servants reverence her dust.

Heathens shall hear and fear thy name,
All kings of earth thy glory know
When thou shalt build up Zion's fame
And live in glory there below.
He'll not despise their prayers, though mute,
But still regard the destitute.

John Clare (based on Psalm 102)

Psalm 40

80

I waited patiently for the LORD;
    he inclined to me and heard my
       cry.
He drew me up from the desolate
       pit,
    out of the miry bog,
and set my feet upon a rock,
    making my steps secure.
He put a new song in my mouth,
    a song of praise to our God.
Many will see and fear,
    and put their trust in the LORD.

81

Lord Jesus,
as you bowed your head and died,
a great darkness covered the land.

We lay before you
the despair of all
who find life
without meaning or purpose,
and see no value in themselves,
who suffer the anguish
of inner darkness
that can only lead them
to self-destruction and death.

Lord,
in your passion, you too
felt abandoned, isolated, derelict.

You are one
with all who suffer
pain and torment
of body and mind.

Be to them the light
that has never been mastered.
Pierce the darkness
which surrounds and engulfs them,
so that they may know
within themselves
acceptance, forgiveness, and peace.

We pray for those who,
through the suicide
of one close to them,
suffer the emptiness of loss
and the burden of untold guilt.

May they know
your gift of acceptance,
so that they may be freed
from self-reproach
and mutual recrimination,
and find in the pattern
of your dying and rising,
new understanding, and purpose
for their lives.

Neville Smith

———⊃⊂———

Cry aloud to the Lord!   82
   O wall of daughter Zion!
Let tears stream down like a
      torrent
   day and night!
Give yourself no rest,
   your eyes no respite!

Arise, cry out in the night,
   at the beginning of the watches!
Pour out your heart like water
   before the presence of the Lord!
Lift your hands to him
   for the lives of your children,
who faint for hunger
   at the head of every street.

The Book of Lamentations

———⊃⊂———

83

Psalm 107

O give thanks to the LORD, for he
is good;
for his steadfast love endures
forever.
Let the redeemed of the LORD say
so,
those he redeemed from trouble
and gathered in from the lands,
from the east and from the
west,
from the north and from the
south.

Some wandered in desert wastes,
finding no way to an inhabited
town;
hungry and thirsty,
their soul fainted within them.
Then they cried to the LORD in
their trouble,
and he delivered them from
their distress;
he led them by a straight way,
until they reached an inhabited
town.
Let them thank the LORD for his
steadfast love,
for his wonderful works to
humankind.
For he satisfies the thirsty,
and the hungry he fills with
good things.

Some sat in darkness and in
 gloom,
  prisoners in misery and in irons,
for they had rebelled against the
 words of God,
  and spurned the counsel of the
  Most High.
Their hearts were bowed down
 with hard labour;
  they fell down, with no one to
  help.
Then they cried to the LORD in
 their trouble,
  and he saved them from their
  distress;
he brought them out of darkness
 and gloom,
  and broke their bonds asunder.
Let them thank the LORD for his
 steadfast love,
  for his wonderful works to
  humankind.
For he shatters the doors of
 bronze,
  and cuts in two the bars of iron.

Some were sick through their
 sinful ways,
  and because of their iniquities
  endured affliction;
they loathed any kind of food,
 and they drew near to the gates
 of death.

Then they cried to the LORD in
their trouble,
and he saved them from their
distress;
he sent out his word and healed
them,
and delivered them from
destruction.
Let them thank the LORD for his
steadfast love,
for his wonderful works to
humankind.
And let them offer thanksgiving
sacrifices,
and tell of his deeds with songs
of joy.

84 Lord Jesus Christ, who for love of our souls entered the deep darkness of the cross, we pray that your healing love may surround all
who are in the darkness of great mental distress and who find it difficult to pray for themselves. May they know that darkness and light
are both alike to you and that you have promised never to fail them
or forsake them.

Llewellyn Cumings

85 Blessed are those who mourn, for
they will be comforted.

The Beatitudes, Gospel of Matthew

Jesus, our brother and friend,
look with kindness and compassion
on those who were sexually abused.
You see the lost child within
still crying alone in the darkness
where the hidden wounds of childhood
still hurt, and make them afraid.
When they feel abandoned, give them hope,
when they feel ashamed, give them comfort,
when they feel unloved, give them faith,
when they feel betrayed, give them peace.
In the power of your resurrection
may love triumph over fear,
light shine in the darkness,
and the long reign of terror be ended.

Tracy Hansen

Chronic Illness and Disability

God of love, whose compassion never fails, we bring before thee the   87
troubles and perils of people and nations, the sighing of prisoners
and captives, the sorrows of the bereaved, the necessities of
strangers, the helplessness of the weak, the despondency of the
weary, the failing powers of the aged. O Lord, draw near to each,
for the sake of Jesus Christ our Lord.

Anselm of Canterbury

⸺◦⸺

When there is no energy left   88
when all has been seen and done
we know that you call us
to let go.

When rest is greatest peace
when sleep is deepest comfort
we know that you call us
to let go.

You call your servant to renewal
you call your servant to find hope.
May we know your gift of life
brings strength we need.

Teach us to let go.

Lisa Withrow

⸺◦⸺

89 Liberating God,
hear our prayers for people who are oppressed today,
as you heard the cries of your people enslaved in Egypt
and raised up Moses to lead them to freedom.

Walk with people who are:

coming out of long-stay psychiatric hospitals
unsure of their place and their welcome
in the communities where they want to live;

coming out of prison after long sentences
unsure of their ability to break the pattern
of former behaviour and association;

coming out of the darkness after years of anguish,
rejection and open hostility and learning not to be
ashamed to be lesbian or gay;

coming through the bleakness of giving up drugs or alcohol
unsure of their ability to face life without these supports;

coming through the waters of grief and loss
unsure of their ability to live alone.

Walk with all who counsel and support them . . .

Walk with all who were once enslaved on their journey to freedom.
Say to them through us, 'I will be your God and I will make you
my people.'

Jean Mortimer

O heavenly Father,
we pray for those suffering from diseases
    for which there is at present no cure.
Give them the victory of trust and hope,
that they may never lose their faith
    in your loving purpose.
Grant your wisdom to all
    who are working to discover the causes of disease,
and the realization that through you
    all things are possible.
We ask this in the name of him
    who went about doing good
    and healing all manner of sickness,
even your Son, Jesus Christ, our Lord.

90

George Appleton

———◦◦———

Holy God, strong Father, nursing Mother,
Jesus, Christ of God, through whom we are sons and
daughters,
reach within us and bring to birth
strength for today and hope for tomorrow.
Hold us in the cradle of your love.
Spirit of God, soothing balm of heaven, may the loss
of childbearing not limit your God-bearing presence
within the sanctuary of our lives.

91

Althea Hayton

———◦◦———

92 Father of compassion and mercy, who never failest to help and
comfort those who cry to thee for succour: give strength and
courage to this thy son in his hour of need. Hold thou him up and
he shall be safe; enable him to feel that thou art near, and to know
that underneath are the everlasting arms; and grant that, resting on
thy protection, he may fear no evil, since thou art with him;
through Jesus Christ our Lord.

Church of Ireland. Book of Common Prayer

93 We beseech thee, Master, to be our helper and protector. Save the
afflicted among us; have mercy on the lowly; raise up the fallen;
appear to the needy; heal the ungodly; restore the wanderers of thy
people; feed the hungry; ransom our prisoners; raise up the sick;
comfort the faint-hearted.

Clement of Rome

94   Dear Lord Jesus,
I don't know who I am,
I don't know what I am,
I don't know where I am,
but please love me.

Prayer of a woman suffering from Alzheimer's Disease

THE DISABLED

God our Father, we offer you thanks and praise for life and all its
blessings:
> the world of sight and sound, touch and taste and smell;
> the gift of language, the power to communicate with others and
> share our thoughts with them;
> the ties of family life and of friendship, in which giving and
> receiving become one and the same;
> the beacon of high ideals;
> and above all for the sense of eternal things amid all that changes,
> and for hope which dares to stretch out beyond the confines
> of this mortal life.

Father, all these things you give, but not everyone has all of them.
In the name of Jesus who went about doing good and making men
and women whole, we pray now for those who are blind or deaf or
dumb. For the paralysed in body, and the isolated in mind. For those
who have no one to trust, and who feel there is no one to trust and
love them. We pray for all whom force of circumstance condemns
to half-life: and for those also whose worst enemy is themselves.

All this we see, and yet there is so much we do not see. Our prej-
udices distort our vision and make our judgments shallow. Keep
restoring our sight, so that we see people in their own right, and
not just for the good or harm they may do us.

Caryl Micklem

Dear Lord, I pray for the innocent babies who are handicapped.
They may feel out of place, rejected and not wanted, but through
friends and adults show them that you really love them, Lord, so
that they grow knowing you faithfully. Through Christ, I pray.

Kigezi diocese, Uganda

97

Blessed are you who take time
to listen to defective speech,
for you help us to know that
if we persevere, we can be
understood.

Blessed are you who walk with
us in public places and ignore
the stares of strangers, for in
your companionship we find
havens of relaxation.

Blessed are you that never bids
us 'hurry up' and more blessed
are you that do not snatch our tasks
from our hands to do them for us,
for often we need time rather than help.

Blessed are you who stand beside
us as we enter new ventures, for
our failures will be outweighed
by times we surprise
ourselves and you.

Blessed are you when by all these
things you assure us that the
thing that makes us individuals
is not our peculiar muscles,
nor our wounded nervous system,
but is the God-given self
that no infirmity can
confine.

Marjorie Chappell

AIDS

Blessed are you, our God, for in Jesus you show us the image of 98
your glory. We give thanks for the gospel of healing and liberation
which is preached to the whole Church in the ministry of those
with HIV or AIDS. May we recognize that it is the real body of
Christ which suffers at this time through HIV and AIDS. It is the
real mind of Christ which is racked by fear and confusion. It is the
real image of God in Christ which is blasphemed in prejudice,
oppression and poverty. May we see in this crisis, loving God, not
punishment but the place where God is most powerfully at work in
Jesus Christ, and where, as sisters and brothers, we can lead each
other to life in all its fullness, given in the same Christ our Lord.

Catholic AIDS Link

We pray for those who are already victims of AIDS, that they may 99
not be led into despair but instead draw nearer to you, commit their
lives into your loving hands and know your loving care. We pray for
the many orphans who are left behind by victims of AIDS, that they
may have hope in you and trust that you will be all in all for them.
We pray this in the name of our Father, Son and Holy Spirit.

Marion Sebuhinja

100 Loving God, you show yourself to those who are vulnerable and make your home with the poor and weak of this world.

Warm our hearts with the fire of your Spirit. Help us to accept the challenges of AIDS.

Protect the healthy, calm the frightened, give courage to those in pain, comfort the dying and give to the dead eternal life.

Console the bereaved, strengthen those who care for the sick.

May we your people, using all our energy and imagination, and trusting in your steadfast love, be united with one another in conquering all disease and fear.

Terrence Higgins Trust Interfaith Group

101 Almighty God, creator of life, sustainer of every good thing I know, my partner with me in the pain of this earth, hear my prayer as I am in the midst of separation and alienation from everything I know to be supportive and healing and true.

AIDS has caused me to feel separated from you. I say, 'Why me? What did I do to deserve this?' . . . Help me to remember that you do not punish your creation by bringing disease, but that you are Emmanuel, God with us. You are as close to me as my next breath.

AIDS has caused a separation between the body I knew and my body now . . . Help me to remember that I am more than my body, and while it pains me greatly to see what has happened to it, I am more than my body . . . I am part of you and you me.

AIDS has separated me from my family . . . O God, help me and them to realize that I haven't changed, I'm still their child, our love for each other is your love for us . . . Help them to overcome their fear, embarrassment and guilt . . . Their love brought me into this world . . . Help them to share as much as possible with me.

AIDS has caused a separation between me and my friends; my friendships have been so important to me. They are especially important now. . . Help me, oh God, to recognize their fear and my increasing need for them to love in any way they can.

AIDS has separated me from society, my whole world and my community. . . It pains me for them to see me differently now . . . Forgive them for allowing their ignorance of this disease and their fear to blind their judgments . . . Help me deal with my anger towards them.

AIDS has caused a separation between me and my church . . . Help the Church restore its ministry to 'the least of these' by reaching out to me and others . . . Help them suspend their judgments and love me as they have before. Help me and them to realize that the Church is the body of Christ . . . that separation and alienation wound the body.

God of my birth and God of my death, help me to know you have been, you are, and you are to come.

Kenneth South

ADDICTION

102 We commend to the care and mercy of our Lord Jesus Christ all who have fallen into the power of substances which cause ruin and misery.

We pray for all those who feel that the 'real world' is so frightening that it must be obliterated by means of alcohol or drugs.

We pray for all who resort to the use of alcohol to cover their inadequacy in facing the demands of life; for those who are so unhappy that they seek a false jollity through heavy drinking.

We commend to the love of God those people, particularly young people, who are slaves to drugs, which stimulates the senses or depress the mind. For those who are now addicts, we pray that they may not lose all hope or sense of reality.

We bring to the Lord, in our prayers, all those who work with the frightened people of our society: alcoholics and their families, those fighting against addiction, and those who have given up the fight.

We pray for those who work in drug addiction units, for doctors, psychiatrists and social workers; and for those who give themselves to such a caring.

We ask the Lord to give each one of us the vision and the strength to live as the free 'slaves of God'; acknowledging the liberty which this gives to us and showing, by our lives, the joy and fulfilment this brings. Through Jesus Christ our Lord.

Church Army

O blessed Jesus, you ministered to all who came to you. Look with 103 compassion upon all who through addiction have lost their health and freedom. Restore to them the assurance of your unfailing mercy; remove the fears that attack them; strengthen them in the work of their recovery; and to those who care for them, give patient understanding and persevering love; for your mercy's sake.

Anglican Church of Canada. Alternative Service Book

For the one who is hurting,
we cry to you, O Healing One.
For the one who is wondering,
we cry to you, O Revealing One.
For the one who is not safe,
we cry to you, O Protecting One.
For the one who faces the unknown,
we cry to you, O Discerning One.
For the one who can be healed
we cry to you, O Suffering One.

Grant this one light for body and mind.
Grant this one a friend in you.
Grant this one strength of support.
Grant this one courage for change.
Grant this one relief from isolation.
Grant this one freedom from bondage.
Grant this one healing of heart and soul.

In your wisdom, we cry to you, O Comforter of the Suffering.

Lisa Withrow

For the inner tyranny
based on outer expectation
of 'acceptable' body, mind and soul,
we repent, O God.

For the one who was not free
from messages all round, speaking
of 'acceptable' body, mind and soul,
we pray, O God.

For the one who heard inner words
that cried 'unacceptable'
we ask your unconditional love, O God.

For those of us left behind,
we pray in our emptiness
we pray in our grief
we pray we might address this injustice
that takes young and old needlessly.
We ask for your forgiveness, your comfort.
We ask that we may know your grace and love.

Lisa Withrow

Illness in Old Age

Lord, support us all the day long of this troublous life, until the   106
shades lengthen and the evening comes and the busy world is
hushed, the fever of life is over and our work is done. Then, Lord,
in your mercy grant us safe lodging, a holy rest and peace at the last;
through Jesus Christ our Lord.

Alternative Service Book (1980)

O Lord Jesus Christ, who didst hear the prayer of thy two disciples   107
and didst abide with them at eventide: Abide, we pray thee, with all
thy people in the evening of life. Make thyself known to them, and
let thy light shine upon their path; and whenever they shall pass
through the valley of the shadow of death, be with them unto the
end; through Jesus Christ our Lord.

George Appleton

Eternal God, we rejoice in your promise that as our day is, so shall   108
our strength be; and we ask your help for all who are old and
wearied with the burden of life. In your strength may they find
courage and peace; and in their advancing years may they learn
more of your love; through Jesus Christ our Lord.

New Every Morning

109 I ask your compassion on one who is groping, like a traveller, through a thick fog of confusion. Remembering the quick spirit, the purposeful activity of this person in former years, we who love him come to you in sorrow. May those who take care of him have patience, gentleness, and perception. If it be your will, restore him to the recognition of people and life around him. If this is not to be, grant that his spirit may be untroubled and that his dreams may be sweet. With our love we commend this dear soul to you.

Josephine Robertson

110   God of mercy,
         look kindly on your servant
         who has grown weak under the burden of years.
         In this holy anointing
         he asks for healing in body and soul.
         Fill him with the strength of your Holy Spirit.
         Keep him firm in faith and serene in hope,
         so that he may give us all an example of patience
         and joyfully witness to the power of your love.
         We ask this through Christ our Lord.

         John Gunstone

When the signs of age begin to mark my body (and still more when   111
they touch my mind); when the ill that is to diminish me or carry
me off strikes from without or is born within me; when the painful
moment comes in which I suddenly awaken to the fact that I am
ill or growing old; and above all at that last moment when I feel I
am losing hold of myself and am absolutely passive within the hands
of the great unknown forces that have formed me; in all those dark
moments, O God, grant that I may understand that it is you (provided only my faith is strong enough) who are painfully parting the
fibres of my being in order to penetrate to the very marrow of my
substance and bear me away within yourself.

Teilhard de Chardin

Losing a Child

O Lord, I felt such terrible disappointment and sadness when they 112 told me my baby had died. I felt so different from all the other mothers. He had been part of my body for all those months, and now he is gone. I wanted to hold him, to feel his warm body in my arms. I wanted to love him. I never had a chance to tell him how much I loved him. I have only cried for him, missing him.

And then I thought of you Lord. I knew he was safe with you. You will love him in such a special way, you will care for him in your heaven. I feel he is safe, Lord. I still miss him, and sometimes when I am alone I cry for him and long for him. But that terrible loneliness is not there when I think that he is at home with you.

Ann Murphy

—◦—

O Lord, there are some women who are crying for not having chil- 113 dren; some of them have had an accident or had an abortion. They badly needed children; they do not show their sorrow to everybody but their hearts are burning with that desire. Help them, Lord, hear their cry. Change their sorrow into happiness. O Lord, listen to our prayers.

Byumba diocese, Rwanda

—◦—

Heavenly Father, by your mighty power you gave us life, and in 114 your love you have given us a new life in Christ Jesus. With these flowers, we remember the tiny new lives these women carried for so short a time. As they lay these flowers close to the light of your presence, may each one of them feel able to lay down the memories of the babies they never saw and their hopes and dreams of parenthood. We ask this in the name of Christ our Lord.

Althea Hayton, Meredith Wheeler and Mrs Cox

—◦—

115   Expecting life,
we now know death;
may we know more than death, O God.
Expecting joy,
we now know pain;
may we know more than pain, O God.
Expecting love,
we now know emptiness;
may we know more than emptiness, O God.
Expecting hope,
we now know despair;
may we know more than despair, O God.
Receive this child in your care,
bless this child whom we barely knew,
renew our faith
renew our hope:
   be with us in our grief, O God.

Lisa Withrow

116 O God we pray that you have mercy on women who have had recurrent miscarriages and stillbirths, that your healing miracle might bring joy into such homes. We pray in the name of Jesus Christ, our Lord.

Mrs A. M. Osaji, Kwara diocese, Nigeria

Lord Jesus, your mother Mary stood by when you were
dying.
Be near to the mothers of these children.
Be to them a strong and loving friend.
Give them healing for hurt,
and hope in place of desperation,
for you alone can show us how
to triumph over death.

Althea Hayton

117

To have known life within
Is to have known joy
And the freshness of beginnings;
To have life snatched away
Leaves me with hands outstretched
My arms open wide,
Feeling emptiness and space
Rather than the weight of my child,
With newborn warmth and silken hair.
My body,
So full of kicks and squirms one day,
Is barren and lifeless the next –
Stripped of its child,
That I never knew.
Yet I did know
And loved.

Judy Gordon Morrow

118

119 Father, help us to entrust this baby N. to your never failing care. We give back to you, our heavenly Father, what you once gave to us; which was always yours and always will be. We believe that we are united with N. in your unending love, through Jesus Christ our Redeemer.

Althea Hayton

———⊃⊂———

120 Heavenly Father, whose Son our Saviour
took little children into his arms and blessed them;
receive, we pray, your child (name) in your never-failing care
   and love,
comfort all who have loved him on earth,
and bring us all to your everlasting kingdom;
through Jesus Christ our Lord.

Prayer at the funeral of a child

———⊃⊂———

Death and Bereavement

I have desired to go
　　Where springs not fail,
To fields where flies no sharp and sided hail
　　And a few lilies blow.

And I have asked to be
　　Where no storms come,
Where the green swell is in the havens dumb,
　　And out of the swing of the sea.

Gerard Manley Hopkins

121

⸺◦⸺

Go forth, O Christian soul, from this world in the name of God the
Father almighty, who created thee; in the name of Jesus Christ, the
Son of the living God, who suffered for thee; in the name of the
Holy Ghost, who was poured out upon thee . . . Today let thy place
be in peace and thine abode holy Sion, through the same Jesus
Christ our Lord.

From the commendation of a soul, Western Rite

122

⸺◦⸺

Lord grant that my last hour
may be my best hour.

Old English prayer

123

⸺◦⸺

124   Lives are woven so intricately together
and death comes unexpectedly, tearing the weave.
In the time of tearing
we pray for your gift of grace, your gift of peace.

For our loved one who travelled in the depths –
    new hope
for our loved one who could not see light –
    bright light
for our loved one who felt alone –
    pure love
for our loved one who preferred to die –
    pure grace.

In the time of tearing
we call for your forgiveness, for your care,
for we did not hear until too late,
for we did not see the valley where our loved one travelled.
In the time of grief,
in the time of confusion,
in the time of guilt,
grant your mercy, your steadfast mercy, we pray.

Lisa Withrow

125   Lord, if I have to die
Let me die;
But please, take away this fear.

Ken Walsh

O my most blessed and glorious creator, that hast fed me all my life   126
long, and redeemed me from all evil; seeing it is thy merciful pleasure to take me out of this frail body, and to wipe away all tears from
mine eyes, and all sorrows from my heart, I do with all humility and
willingness consent and submit myself wholly unto thy sacred will.
My most loving redeemer, into thy saving and everlasting arm I
commend my spirit; I am ready, my dear Lord, and earnestly expect
and long for thy good pleasure. Come quickly, and receive the soul
of thy servant which trusteth in thee.

Henry Vaughan

God our heavenly Father, Lord of peace, God of love, we pray you   127
guide all children who have lost their parents and are living in hard
times. Lead them in everything they do, send your love into the
hearts of those caring for them. Let this group know your love for
them and they will praise you.

Penina Tito Bazia

Bring us, O Lord our God, at our last awakening into the house and   128
gate of heaven, to enter into that gate and dwell in that house,
where there shall be no darkness or dazzling, but one equal light;
no noise or silence, but one equal music; no fears or hopes, but one
equal possession; no ends or beginnings, but one equal eternity; in
the habitations of thy glory and dominion world without end.

John Donne

129 O Lord, you have freed us from the fear of death. You have made the end of our life here into the beginning of true life for us. You give rest to our bodies for a time in sleep, and then you awaken them again with the sound of the last trumpet. Our earthly body, formed by your hands, you consign in trust to the earth, and then once more you reclaim it, transfiguring with immortality and grace whatever in us is mortal or deformed. You have opened for us the way to resurrection, and given to those that fear you the sign of the holy cross as their emblem, to destroy the enemy and to save our life.

Eternal God, on you have I depended from my mother's womb, you have I loved with all the strength of my soul, to you have I dedicated my flesh and my soul from my youth until now. Set by my side an angel of light, to guide me to the place of repose, where are the waters of rest, among the holy Fathers. You have broken the fiery sword and restored to Paradise the thief who was crucified with you and implored your mercy: remember me also in your kingdom, for I too have been crucified with you. Let not the dread abyss separate me from your elect. Let not the envious one bar the way before me. But forgive me and accept my soul into your hands, spotless and undefiled, as incense in your sight.

Macrina, fourth century

130 We bring before you, O Lord Christ, those whose earthly life is almost at an end. Lessen their fear, encourage them on their journey and give them the peace that comes from your victory over death.

Author unknown

O Lord God, this loss hurts so. My dead are so alive, I cannot believe   131
I cannot touch them or speak to them. I so want them, Father, so
miss them . . . I *bleed*, Father. Help me; help me in this fog, which
blots out my perspective on the life they now live in your hereafter.
Give me hope, dear Lord God, give me hope in Christ's own defeat
of death, that one day I shall see my loved ones again; and touch
them and hear them, not in the vividness of my mind's eye; not in
dreams or memories; but in that world of light to which, O my loving Lord, safely bring me.

Ruth Etchells

Let not mistaken mercy   132
blind my fading sight,
no false euphoria lull me.
I would not unprepared
take this last journey.
Give me a light to guide me
through dark valleys,
a staff to lean upon,
bread to sustain me,
a blessing in my ear
that fear may not assail me.
Then leaving do not hold my hand,
I go to meet a friend –
     that same who traced
     compassion in the sand.

Nancy Hopkins

133 We give back to you, O God, those whom you gave to us. You did not lose them when you gave them to us and we do not lose them by their return to you.

Your dear Son has taught us that life is eternal and love cannot die, so death is only an horizon and an horizon is only the limit of our sight. Open our eyes to see more clearly and draw us close to you that we may know that we are nearer to our loved ones, who are with you. You have told us that you are preparing a place for us; prepare us also for that happy place, that where you are we may also be always, O dear Lord of life and death.

William Penn

————⊂⊃————

134   God of the dark night,
                you were with Jesus praying in the garden,
                you were with Jesus all the way to the cross
                and through the resurrection.
            Help us to recognize you now,
                as we watch with our friend,
                and wait for what must happen;
                help us through any bitterness and despair,
                help us accept our distress,
                help us to remember that you care for us
                and that in your will is our peace.

Anglican Church in Aotearoa and Polynesia.
A New Zealand Prayer Book

————⊂⊃————

O God, our heavenly Father, who does not want us, your children, 135
to be in sorrow, come down now and be with our brothers and sisters who have lost their husbands/wives. Comfort them during
their hard times, when they are alone at night or day; be with them
to encourage and strengthen them. May they pass their days here on
earth in the assurance that they will join you in your heavenly kingdom where there will be no more sorrow, weeping and pain.

Rhoda Ade Olarewaju

We remember, Lord, the slenderness of the thread which separates 136
life from death, and the suddenness with which it can be broken.
Help us also to remember that on both sides of that division we are
surrounded by your love.

Persuade our hearts that when our dear ones die neither we nor
they are parted from you.

In you may we find peace, and in you be united with them in
the body of Christ, who has burst the bonds of death and is alive
for evermore, our Saviour and theirs for ever and ever.

Dick Williams

If I should go before the rest of you 137
Break not a flower, nor inscribe a stone.
Nor talk of me in a Sunday voice;
But be the usual selves that I have known.
   Weep if you must, parting is hell;
   But life goes on – so sing as well.

Joyce Grenfell

138

O God, give me of thy wisdom,
O God, give me of thy mercy,
O God, give me of thy fulness,
And of thy guidance in face of every strait.

O God, give me of thy holiness,
O God, give me of thy shielding,
O God, give me of thy surrounding,
And of thy peace in the knot of my death.

O give me of thy surrounding,
And of thy peace at the hour of my death!

Source unknown (Celtic)

139　In my grief, numb and empty I come. I come to give the burden I cannot feel; I cannot feel, for to feel is now too much. Too much, for my heart's too full, too full of anger and unshed tears.

Lord, you wept, knew anger and what it is to feel alone. Let my tears spill over to fill the void of loneliness, of being on my own. Help me to remember the good times, link me with those who know this place I'm in.

Empty I come, to be filled with my tears and your love.

Rochester diocese, England

O Lord God, who knowest our frame and rememberest that we are 140
dust, look in pity upon those who mourn. Make thy loving presence so real to them that they may feel round about them thine everlasting arms, upholding and strengthening them.

Grant them such a sense of certainty that their loved one is with thee, doing thy high service, unhindered by pain, that they may turn to life's tasks with brave hearts and steady nerves, consoled in the thought that they will meet their dear one again.

Teach us all to face death unafraid and take us at last in triumph through the shadows into thine everlasting light where are reunion and never-ending joy. Through Jesus Christ our Lord.

Leslie D. Weatherhead

As thou wast before 141
At my life's beginning,
Be thou so again
At my journey's end.

As thou wast beside
At my soul's shaping,
Father, be thou too
At my journey's close.

Scots Celtic prayer

SUBJECT INDEX

INDEX OF AUTHORS
AND SOURCES

ACKNOWLEDGEMENTS

Permission to use the following prayers has been kindly granted by the copyright holders. We made our best endeavour to track all sources, but if we are told of any errors or omissions, these will be corrected at reprint.

Adam, David, from *Tides and Seasons* (Triangle, 1989) 6

The Anglican Church in Aotearoa, New Zealand and Polynesia, from *A New Zealand Prayer Book – He Karakia Mihinare o Aotearoa* 134

The Anglican Church of Canada, from *The Book of Alternative Services* of the Anglican Church of Canada, copyright © 1985 by the General Synod of the Anglican Church of Canada 103

Appleton, George, adapted by Jim Cotter, from Jim Cotter, *Prayer at Night: A Book for the Darkness* (Cairns Publications, 1983) 15; Appleton, George, from George Appleton (compiler), *Acts of Devotion*. 2nd Revised Edition (SPCK, 1963) 90

Archbishops' Council The Church of England, from *The Alternative Service Book 1980*, copyright © The Archbishops' Council 106, 120

Augsburg Fortress Press, from Leslie F. Brandt, *Book of Christian Prayer*, copyright © 1974 Augsburg Publishing House 32

BBC Publications, from *New Every Morning*. New Edition (1973), copyright © British Broadcasting Corporation, 1973 40, 108

Cambridge University Press, from *The Book of Common Prayer*, the rights in which are vested in the Crown, reprinted by permission of the Crown's Patentee, Cambridge University Press 41, 48

Canterbury Press, from *Hymns Ancient & Modern*. New Standard Version (1983) 30

Church Army, from Basil Napier and Michael King (compilers), *Front Line Praying* (1981), copyright © Church Army and BRF, 1981 102

Church Mission Society, from John Carden (editor), *Morning, Noon and Night* (1976) 76

Church of St Marylebone, from Ernest Lucas (editor), *Christian Healing, What can we believe?* (Lynx Communications, 1997) 28, 37

Crescent Moon Publishing, from *Poems* by Henry Vaughan, edited by A. H. Ninham (Joe's Press, 1994) 126

The Crossroad Publishing Co. and HarperCollins Publishers Australia, from Miriam Therese Winter, *Woman Wisdom: A Feminist Lectionary and Psalter: Women of the Hebrew Scriptures: Part One*, copyright © 1991 by Medical Mission Sisters 39

Darton, Longman & Todd Ltd, Orbis Books and St Paul Publications, from Sheila Cassidy, *Good Friday People*, copyright © 1990 Darton, Longman & Todd 42

Epworth Press, from Maureen Edwards (editor), *Living Prayers for Today: An Anthology of Prayers for Many Occasions* (NCEC, 1996) 78

Etchells, Ruth, *Just As I Am* (SPCK, 1994) 131

Furlong, Monica, from *The SPCK Book of Christian Prayer* (1995) 8

Hansen, Tracy, *Seven for a Secret That's Never Been Told* (Triangle, 1991) 86

HarperCollins Publishers Ltd, from Kathy Keay (editor), *Laughter, Silence and Shouting: An Anthology of Women's Prayers* (Marshall Pickering, 1994) 7, 21, 97, 123

Terrence Higgins Trust, from Catherine von Ruhland (editor), *Prayers from the Edge* (Triangle, 1995) 100

Highland Books, from John Gunstone, *Prayers for Healing* (1987), © John Gunstone, 1987 19, 29, 34, 38, 44, 49, 74, 110

Hodder and Stoughton Publishers, from Leslie D. Weatherhead, *A Private House of Prayer* (Arthur James, 1985) 140; from Frank Colquhoun (editor), *God of Our Fathers: Prayers of the British Isles* (Hodder, 1994) 33

The Iona Community, *A Wee Worship Book* (1989), copyright © 1989 Wild Goose Worship Group, The Iona Community 35

Arthur James Press, from Althea Hayton (compiler), *Not Out of Mind* (1998) 52, 59, 91, 114, 117, 119; from Denis Duncan, *A Day at a Time* (1987) 62

Kingsway Publications, from Dick Williams (editor), *More Prayers for Today's Church* (1984) 136

Lion Publishing, from Mary Batchelor (editor), *The Lion Prayer Collection* (1992) 47, 122, 125, 128, 130, 133, 141

McCrimmon Publishing, from Tony Castle (editor), *The Family Book of Prayer* (1988) 107

McIlhagga, Kate, from Kate Compston (editor), *Encompassing Presence*, the Prayer Handbook for 1993 (United Reformed Church, 1992), © Kate McIlhagga, 1992 4

McRae-McMahon, Dorothy, from Dorothy McRae-McMahon, *The Glory of Blood, Sweat and Tears* (Uniting Education, 1993) 22; from Dorothy McRae-McMahon, *Liturgies for the Journeys of Life* (SPCK, 2000) 25, 27

Millar, Peter, from Maureen Edwards (editor), *Living Prayers for Today: An Anthology of Prayers for Many Occasions* (NCEC, 1996) 9

Missionaries of Charity, from Kathryn Spink (editor), *In the Silence of the Heart: Meditations by Mother Teresa* (SPCK, 1983) 46

Mortimer, Jean, *Exceeding our Limits* (URC 1991) 89

Mothers' Union, from Rachel Stowe (compiler), *Women At Prayer: Day-by-Day Prayers for Every Woman* (Marshall Pickering, 1994) 23, 24, 31, 51, 53; 55; 58; 63, 65, 66, 68, 69; 96, 99, 112; 113; 116; 127, 135, 139

National Christian Education Council, from Maureen Edwards (editor), *Living Prayers for Today: An Anthology of Prayers for Many Occasions* (1996) 72; from Henry McKeating (editor), *More Everyday Prayers* (1982) 12; and from David Jenkins (editor), *Further Everyday Prayers* (1987) 50

National Council of the Churches of Christ in the USA, from *New Revised Standard Version of the Bible*, copyright © 1989 by the Division of Christian Education of the National Council of the Churches of Christ in the USA 1, 5, 14, 20, 70, 80, 82, 83, 85

William Neill-Hall Literary Agency, from Mary Batchelor (editor), *The Lion Prayer Collection* (1992), © Mary Batchelor, 1992 56

Thomas Nelson Inc., from Judy Gordon Morrow and Nancy Gordon DeHamer (editors), *Good Mourning* (Word Music & Publishing, 1989) 118

New City Press, from Wolfgang Bader (editor), *Prayers of St Francis* (1994) 64

Oxford University Press, 'Heaven-Haven' from C. Phillips (editor), *Gerard Manley Hopkins* (1986) 121; from Neville Smith (editor), *Prayers for People in Hospital* (1994) 81; and from *Church of Ireland Book of Common Prayer* (1981) 92